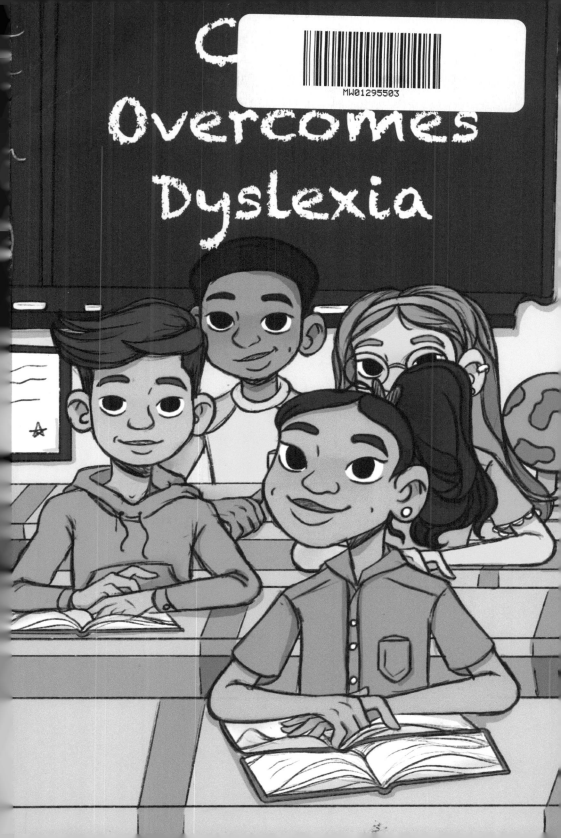

C
Overcomes
Dyslexia

Xulon Press
2301 Lucien Way #415
Maitland, FL 32751
407.339.4217
www.xulonpress.com

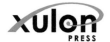

Printed in the United States of America

Paperback ISBN-13: 978-1-6628-0891-3
Ebook ISBN-13: 978-1-6628-0892-0

Carey Overcomes Dyslexia

Written by
Aarian Daniels

Illustrated by
Makayla Perry

XULON PRESS

To my husband and daughters...the journey is never easy but telling the story is amazing. You make me so proud to be your wife and mother. I love you!

To my parents, Aunt Dana, Keith and my in-laws, thank you for your love, support and encouragement.

To the people in my life that make me smile, support, encourage and bring me joy...THANK YOU!

Special thanks to Lauren and Malaika. For always encouraging me and helping to channel my ideas into a reality.

The school year was off to a good start for Carey. She liked her school, her teachers, and her classmates. Each day after school, she and her sister Alle would complete their homework. Alle would finish her work in a breeze, but Carey would often need to ask her mom and dad for help.

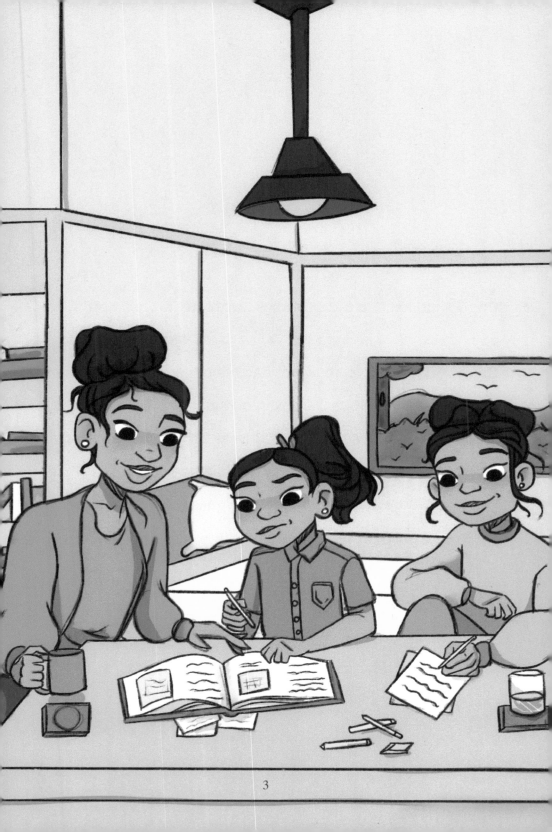

Carey's mother and father always taught her to work hard and do her best. So when the first report cards were sent home, Carey was excited to show her parents her grades. When she and Alle got off the bus Carey ran ahead to show them her report. Her mother started to read what Carey received. Her face was all smiles - A's and B's in all subjects except… reading? Carey noticed her mother's smile fade into a frown. Carey had received a D.

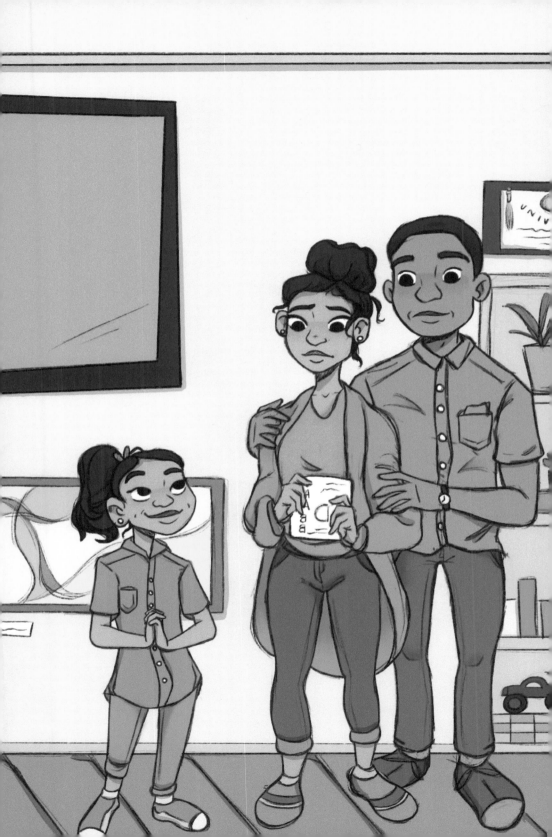

"What's wrong Mommy?" asked Carey.

Carey's mom glanced at the report card, "Are you having trouble in reading?"

"No," said Carey, feeling slightly embarrassed.

"Are you sure?" asked her mom gently.

"Umm, I don't think so…"

"Okay, Carey," said her mom, "Well, you are not in trouble. You and your sister did a great job on your report cards. I am going to call your teacher, Mr. Philips, to see what help you may need."

"Okay, Mommy!" Carey said cheerfully.

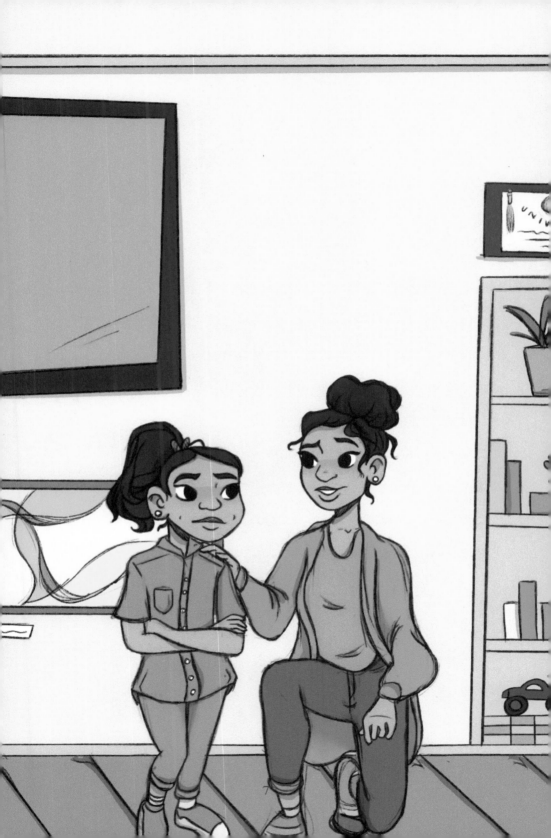

The next day Carey's mom called Mr. Philips to schedule an appointment to talk about her grade in reading. During the meeting, Carey's teacher said that she was a wonderful student, and that she was kind, helpful, and caring to the other students.

"Carey is great," said Mr. Philips.

"She makes us very proud," said her mom smiling.

"And she should," Mr. Philips said. "The only trouble I have with Carey is that she struggles with reading."

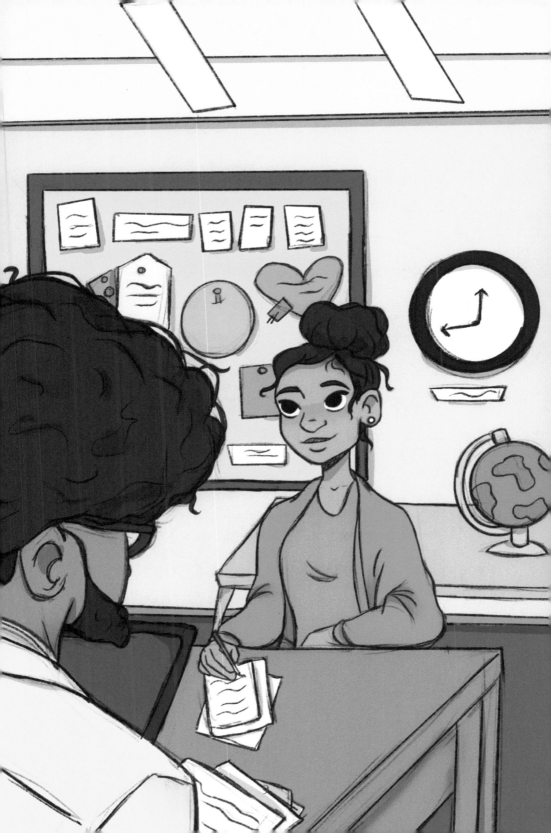

"How does she struggle with reading?" asked Carey's mom, frowning.

"Carey has trouble sounding out her words," said Mr. Philips, "She often mixes up letters and has trouble spelling."

Carey's mom began to replay memories in her head of Carey reading.

"Have you noticed Carey can pronounce a word only after you've said it?" questioned Mr. Philips.

Carey's mom thought of times when Carey struggled while reading with her dad or her sister.

"I know this is hard for you," said Mr. Philips gently, "But I have some suggestions that could help Carey improve her reading."

Carey's mom reached for her cell phone and began to take notes.

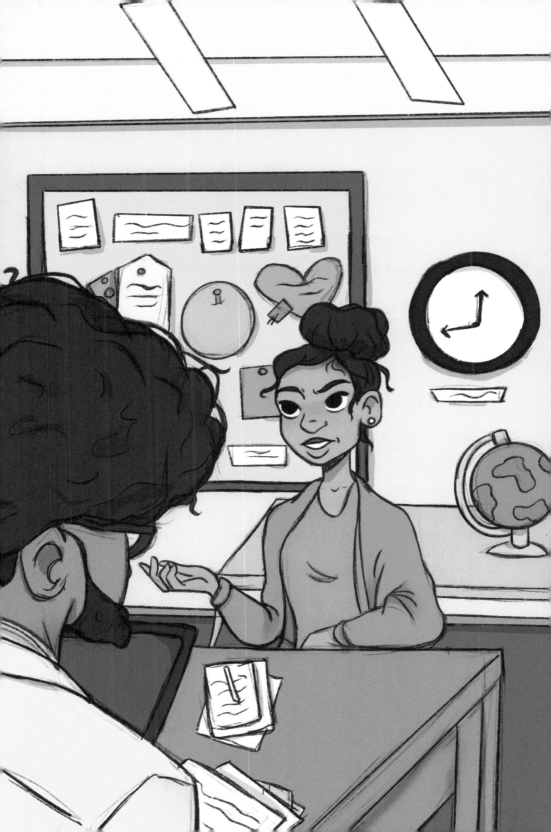

The next grading period came and went, and Carey's grade in reading was even lower than before. She was no longer excited to wake up and go to school and would eat her breakfast as slowly as possible before the bus came. As her schoolwork and homework got harder in reading, Carey struggled even more with reading, spelling, and sounding out words.

"Carey, is school hard for you?" Carey's mom asked on the ride home one afternoon.

"Umm, no," said Carey. "I like school."

"Is reading hard for you?" Carey's mom asked glancing over at Carey staring out the window

"No!" bellowed Carey, blushing. After a few minutes Carey looked up at her mother, sadly.

"Yes, Mommy. Reading is hard for me."

Not wanting their daughter to give up on school, Carey's mom and dad e-mailed Mr. Philips to have another meeting about helping Carey improve her reading skills.

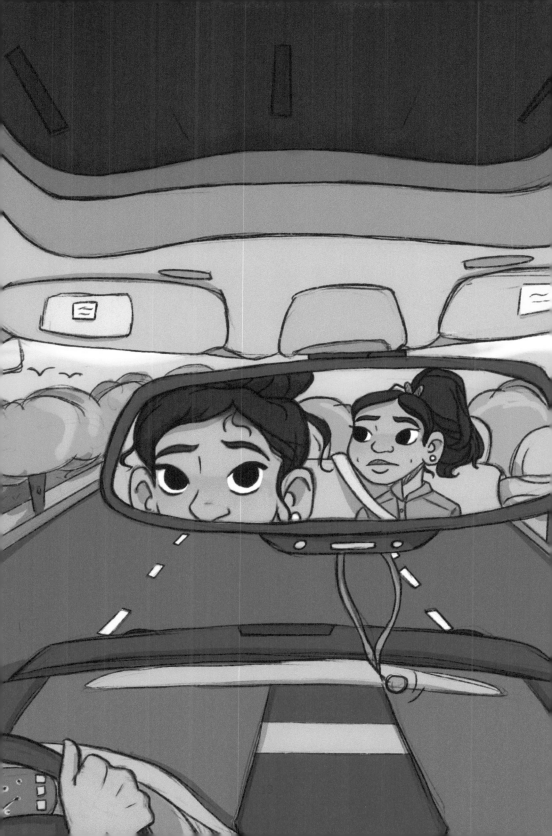

Carey's dad was becoming frustrated. Like Carey's mom, he wasn't sure how to help Carey and felt helpless as he watched her struggle with reading. Seeing his daughter's confidence fade was hard but he was determined to help her get through it. The night before their meeting with Mr. Philips, Carey's dad heard her talking to her favorite stuffed animal, Gichy, in her room. Gichy and Carey were inseparable. If she didn't have her sister Alle to play with, Carey always had Gichy. As Carey was talking to Gichy, tears were rolling down her face.

"Gichy, I try very hard to spell and read, but I can't do it," said Carey between hiccups and tears.

"I try so hard. I don't want Mommy and Daddy to be upset with me." Carey helplessly looked at Gichy, "What can I do?"

As Carey hugged Gichy tightly, her father could see the gold lettering reflecting on the bear's vest:

Glad

I

Can

Help

You

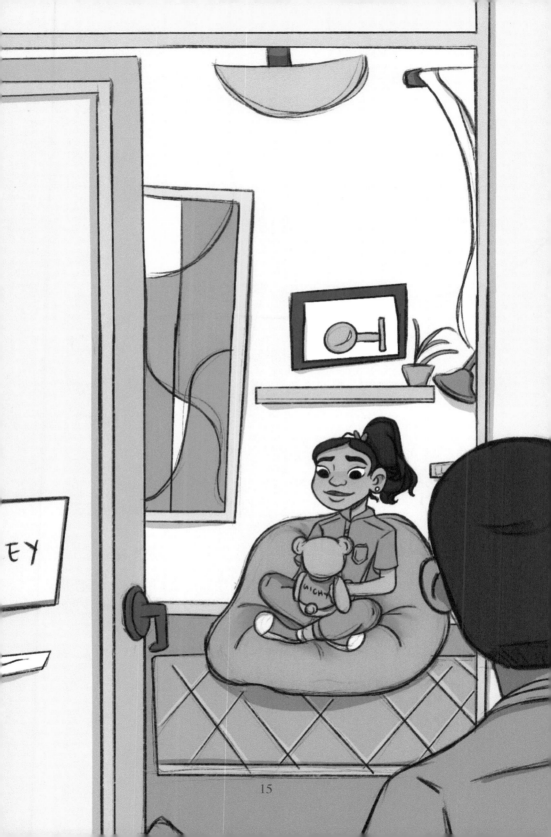

The next morning Carey's mom and dad gave her a big hug. They told her they were going to do all they could to help her and that everything was going be all right.

"We all need help sometimes," Carey's dad said to her. She smiled and gave her parents a big hug back.

Carey's mom and dad dropped them off at school that morning. While she and Alle went to go play with their friends before the first bell, Carey's mom and dad went to talk with Mr. Philips.

"If Carey's grade in reading does not improve, she'll have to stay in the first grade." Mr. Philips told her parents.

"She is trying her hardest, Mr. Philips," pleaded Carey's mom, "Please don't hold her back."

"I don't want to, but she is still having trouble reading," explained Mr. Philips. "However, I do have one more suggestion that could help Carey."

Mr. Philips referred Carey's parents to a reading specialist who determined that Carey had a learning disability called dyslexia.

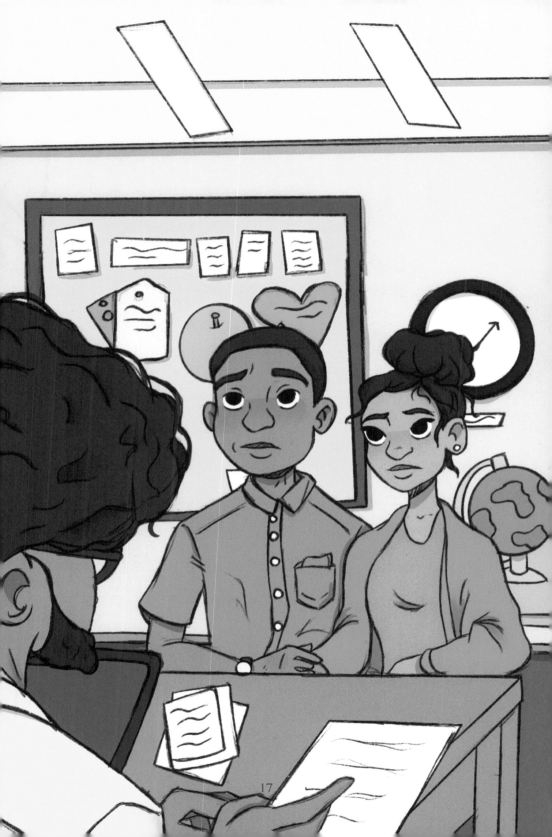

"Is this a bad thing? Am I going to be okay?" asked Carey, her eyes wide.

"Baby, you are going to be just fine," her mom said warmly.

"We now know how to help you, Carey," said her dad with a smile.

"Do I have dyslexia?" asked Alle.

"No, Alle. You do not have it."

"Okay," said Alle. "Well, how did Carey get it?"

"Dyslexia is hereditary," said Carey's mom, "that means our immediate family members do not have it, but this gene has been passed down to Carey. Carey could have gotten it from my side of the family or your father's side of the family."

"But I'm going to be okay - right Mommy?" said Carey grinning.

"Yes," Carey's mom said smiling. "Yes, you are. We're going to get you a reading specialist that can help you with your dyslexia."

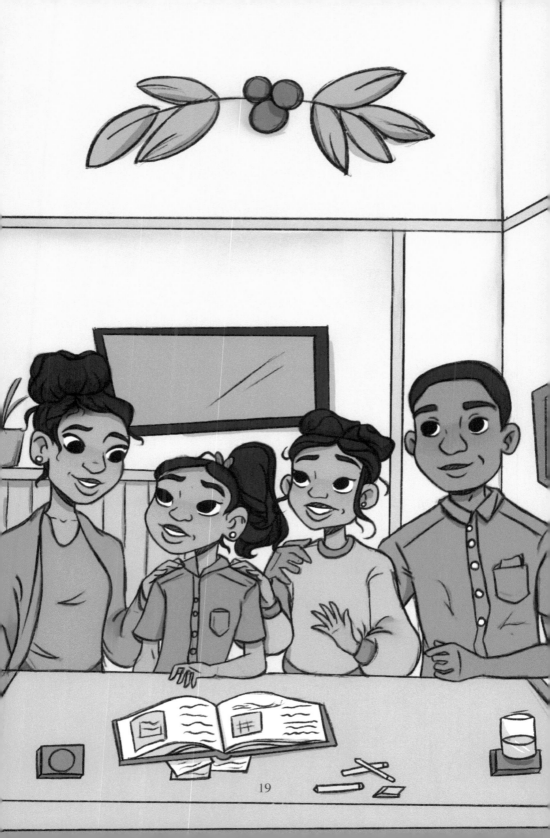

For an hour, three days a week Carey worked with a reading specialist who gave her techniques to manage her dyslexia. At first, it was not easy for Carey to work through her assignments, but she worked very hard despite her frustration. She learned that some of the greatest minds in history, like Albert Einstein, also had dyslexia. Fun arts and crafts projects, like spelling with playdough and painting, helped Carey recognize letters and words by seeing them in a different way. After school, she and Alle would play hopscotch and jump rope to spell out words. Carey also read out loud and used audio resources in school to help her feel more comfortable. Soon her grade in reading improved and she was able to go to second grade!

"Mommy, I did it!" cried Carey, beaming with joy.

"Yes, you did!" her mom beamed back at her. "Baby, you may have dyslexia, but dyslexia does not have you."

"You are right, Mommy," said Carey hugging her mom tightly.

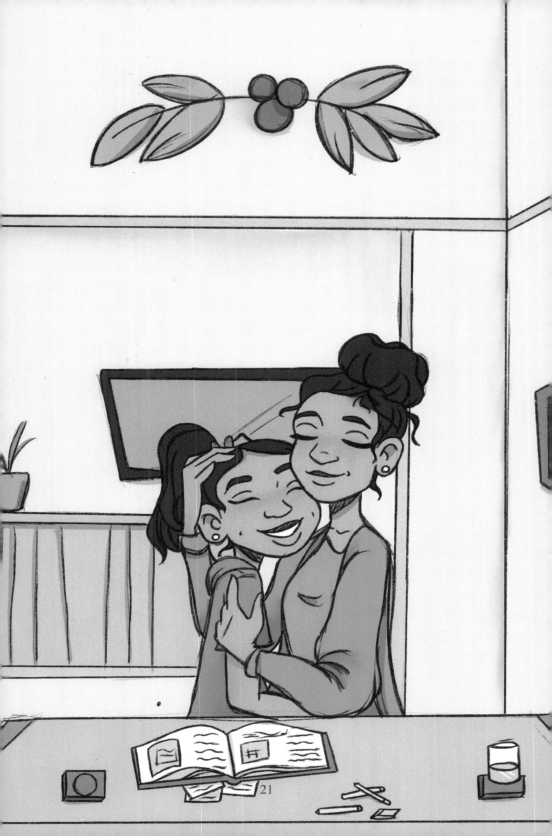

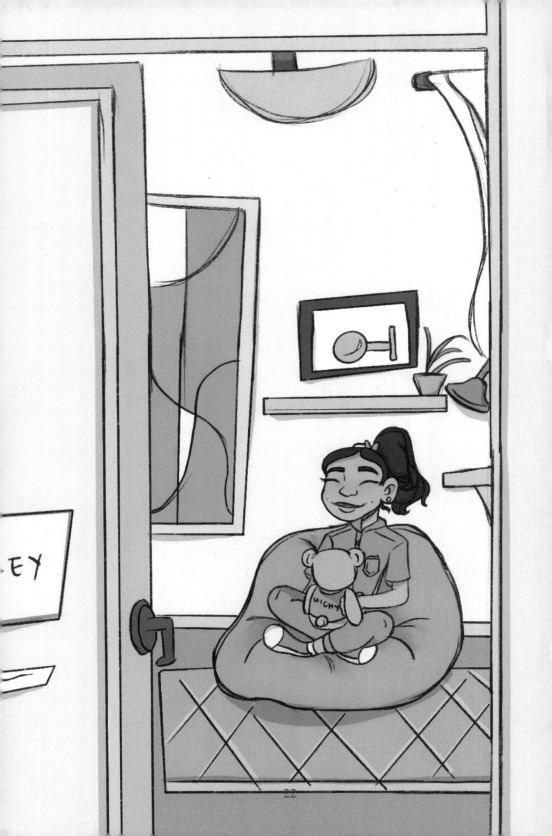

CPSIA information can be obtained
at www.ICGtesting.com
Printed in the USA
BVHW051311300321
603709BV00010B/144